Nour Louati

Regulation of anti-erythrocytic alloimmunization

Nour Louati

Regulation of anti-erythrocytic alloimmunization

Sickle cell disease

ScienciaScripts

Imprint

Any brand names and product names mentioned in this book are subject to trademark, brand or patent protection and are trademarks or registered trademarks of their respective holders. The use of brand names, product names, common names, trade names, product descriptions etc. even without a particular marking in this work is in no way to be construed to mean that such names may be regarded as unrestricted in respect of trademark and brand protection legislation and could thus be used by anyone.

Cover image: www.ingimage.com

This book is a translation from the original published under ISBN 978-620-6-73126-9.

Publisher:
Sciencia Scripts
is a trademark of
Dodo Books Indian Ocean Ltd. and OmniScriptum S.R.L publishing group

120 High Road, East Finchley, London, N2 9ED, United Kingdom
Str. Armeneasca 28/1, office 1, Chisinau MD-2012, Republic of Moldova, Europe
Managing Directors: Ieva Konstantinova, Victoria Ursu
info@omniscriptum.com

Printed at: see last page
ISBN: 978-620-3-24573-8

TABLE OF CONTENTS

Introduction

Sickle cell anaemia is an autosomal recessive haemoglobinopathy which mainly affects people living in the West Indies and Central and North Africa. It is the most widespread haemoglobinopathy in the world(1) . Its incidence in Tunisia is 1.9%(2) . It is characterised by a mutation in the ß globin gene, resulting in the production of an abnormal haemoglobin, haemoglobin S, responsible for the sickling of red blood cells (RBCs) in an oxygen-depleted environment. This abnormal haemoglobin is responsible for the acute and chronic complications of the disease, including haemolytic anaemia, vaso-occlusive crises, strokes, morphine-induced pain, acute chest syndrome and priapism .(3)

Blood transfusion remains a key treatment in the management of this disease. In fact, 60-90% of people with sickle cell disease have received transfusions in the course of their lives(4) . Transfusion is used to reduce haemoglobin S levels and therefore to prevent or treat the complications of this disease, in the form of a simple transfusion or exchange transfusion, either in an acute setting or as part of a long-term transfusion protocol .(5)

The major immunological risk of transfusion is anti-erythrocyte alloimmunisation, which can lead to serious immunohaemolytic reactions, delayed delivery of compatible red blood cells (RBCs) and even transfusion impasse situations.

Alloimmunisation may be expressed either by the acquisition of one or more alloantibodies (Ac) which will make subsequent transfusions difficult, or by an immediate or delayed haemolytic event. In addition, there is a transfusion complication specific to sickle cell disease, which is post-transfusion hyperhaemolysis. Occurring immediately or after a delay, it is defined as a drop in haemoglobin concentration to a value below the pre-transfusion value.

It is secondary to hyperhaemolysis, which also affects autologous red blood cells that are simply "bystanders" to a phenomenon that does not concern them (*stander haemolysis*). The mechanism of hyperhaemolysis has not yet been clearly identified. Irregular antibodies are not always found after such an episode .(6)

This risk alloimmunisation is particularly high in sickle cell disease(7) with a frequency that varies widely from one study to another, ranging from 6 to 35%, with a median of 25%. In our country, alloimmunisation is still a frequent complication in sickle cell patients, with frequencies of 14% in the Sfax region(8) and 16% in the Tunis region .(9)

Some studies have reported higher rates of alloimmunisation in sickle cell disease compared to other conditions requiring multiple transfusions -(911) while others have not found these results - .(1214)

This disparity in alloimmunisation results, whether between sickle cell disease and other pathologies treated by multiple transfusions or within sickle cell disease itself, raises questions about the reasons why sickle cell patients develop higher rates of anti-erythrocyte alloimmunisation and differences in response to erythrocyte antigens (Ag) from one patient to another, which means that we need to take stock of current knowledge on this subject.

We conducted a general review of the literature with a view to gaining a better understanding of the mechanisms regulating alloimmunisation in this highly vulnerable population, and consequently improving risk management by implementing a preventive transfusion strategy wherever possible.

Materials and methods

1. Search strategy

A search of the Pub Med electronic database was carried out to identify the mechanisms by which alloimmunisation is regulated in sickle cell disease patients. The following MeSH terms "regulation or mechanisms or pathophysiology - alloimmunisation - sickle cell disease" were used. The full texts cited up to September 2019 were taken into consideration, as well as most of their references for a broader study.

2. Selection criteria

The choice of articles took into account the following inclusion criteria:

- journals or research articles, including those published in Tunisia,
- alloimmunisation secondary to blood transfusion
- alloimmunisation in sickle cell patients only

3. Data extraction

Two independent reviewers checked each article and extracted the following data from the eligible studies: name of the first author, year publication, country of origin, ethnic origin of the population studied, nature of the alloantibodies detected, frequency and pathophysiology of alloimmunisation, risk factors or mechanisms thought to be involved in alloimmunisation or currently being studied.

Results

Alloimmunisation in sickle cell disease has been detected for over fifty years and remains poorly understood. There are many suggested pathophysiological mechanisms and predisposing factors:

1. Mechanisms of anti-erythrocyte alloimmunisation

Anti-erythrocyte alloimmunisation involves multiple steps including recognition of the Ag present on the donor RBC, processing and presentation of the Ag by the HLA class II system to the T cell receptor (TCR), activation of CD4+ T helper lymphocytes (Ly Th2), interaction of T and B lymphocytes and finally differentiation of B cells into plasma cells (Figure 1).

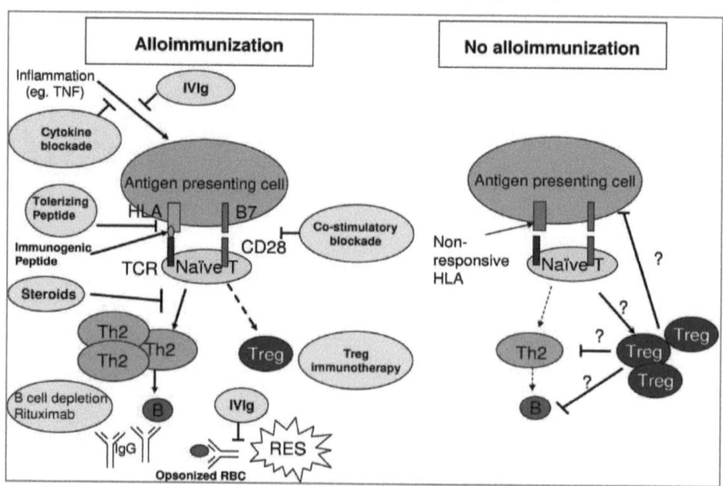

Figure1 : Hypothetical diagram of the immune response to red cell antigens in antigens in allo- and non-alloimmunised patients (25).

Several factors involved in alloimmunisation are described. Preventive actions and specific stages in the prevention of alloimmunisation are shown in yellow. In addition, the modes of action   The hypothetical model predicts that the chronic inflammatory state present in sickle cell disease creates a microenvironment with increased inflammatory cytokines, which favours antigen-presenting cells (APCs), such as macrophages and dendritic cells to increase phagocytosis of transfused RBCs, and also favours the generation of immunogenic peptides by APCs. The patient's HLA repertoire will then dictate whether these peptides are   presented to naive CD4+ T helper (Th) cells or not. In alloimmunised patients, Th2 frequency is increased, which is normally associated with a humoral immune response, and Treg activity is decreased. In sickle cell patients who may have a genetic predisposition not to alloimmunise, the peptides presented by APCs may be less immunostimulatory, so that naive CD4 + cells are tolerant and lead to induction of reg T cells which may decrease Th2 and/or B cells and decrease Treg activity.   Th2 and/or B cells and activate APCs ("?").

Murine and human studies have shown that the process of alloimmunisation to erythrocyte Ag can be modulated at each of these stages by acquired and genetic factors, although the relevance of these factors to alloimmunisation in sickle cell disease has not been fully elucidated.

Antigenic differences between donors and recipients of RGCs are necessary for the initial triggering of alloimmunisation. In sickle cell disease, several studies have shown that the risk of alloimmunisation increases with an increasing number of transfusions .(16–21)

In addition, women have a higher rate of alloimmunisation(21) which partly explained by exposure during pregnancy .(22)

Not all patients develop allo-AC after exposure to a RGC transfusion. This applies not only to patients with sickle cell disease but also to all polytransfusion recipients. A recent mathematical modelling study supported the hypothesis that alloimmunised patients represent a genetically distinct group with increased susceptibility to RBC sensitisation(23) Within this group, only 30% will produce Ac, raising the possibility that recipient factors, including the nature of underlying disease, may influence alloimmunisation in at-risk recipients. Recipients can thus be classified as responders and non-responders.

Currently, many studies have led to a better understanding of these "dependent" recipient mechanisms(23–25) , but there is still a vast field of investigation to fully understand all the factors involved.

2. Factors predisposing to alloimmunisation

A review of the literature revealed numerous factors predisposing sickle cell patients to alloimmunisation.

A distinction is made between factors linked to RGC recipients, i.e. those specific to sickle cell disease, and those linked to the RGC transfused.

2.1. Factors related to the blood donor or the RGC transfused

2.1.1. Type of RGC transfused: phenotyped or standard

Since the systematic use of RH-KEL1 phenotyped RGCs in sickle cell transfusion patients, anti-erythrocyte alloimmunisation has decreased in some countries, since the majority of antibodies (Ac) previously encountered appeared in these systems.

The study by Norol et al. reported a reduction in the prevalence of alloimmunisation in sickle cell patients from 30.6% in the case of transfusion of standard RGCs to 8.2% in the case of phenotyped RGCs(26) . Similarly, in a study of 32 sickle cell children receiving monthly erythrocytopheresis sessions, Grodfey et al. reported a reduction in alloimmunisation rates (from 0.189/100 to 0.053/100) after the use of RGCs compatible with Ag C, E and Kell(27) . In a study carried out at the Sfax regional blood transfusion centre (CRTS) in 54 major sickle cell patients, the study of allo-Ac showed that the majority of them Rhesus and KEL specific and were developed following transfusion of standard RGCs(8) . This was also reported in the study by Nawel et al (8).

Castro et al. have shown that phenotyping in the Rhesus and KEL systems can prevent alloimmunisation in 53% of patients who develop allo-Ac, and in 70% if phenotyping is extended to the Ss, Duffy and Kidd systems(28) . Transfusion of phenotyped RGCs would reduce the risk of alloimmunisation and improve transfusion of patients with sickle cell disease.

2.1.2. Number of RGCs transfused and transfusion episodes

The second factor influencing the risk of alloimmunisation is the cumulative number of red blood cells received. However, this notion has recently been called into question.

Indeed, while some studies have not associated the high rate of alloimmunisation with the number of units transfused or transfusion episodes performed -(7,8,15,2225) and it has even been suggested that the risk of alloimmunisation is minimal after 10 to 20 transfusions(26) and that 50% of immunised patients produce their 1stAc before the 8th transfusion episode(32) , other studies -)(22, 2631 have shown a strong correlation between the prevalence of alloimmunisation and the number of transfusions received. Rosse et al report a risk of alloimmunisation persisting even after transfusion of 50 or 100 units of RGCs in 1814 patients transfused for major sickle cell syndromes(18) . Silvy et al report a 61% risk of producing a new Ac by an immunised patient with each new transfusion .(33)

2.1.3. Immunomodulatory effect of transfusions

Blood transfusion has an immunosuppressive effect, regardless of the underlying pathology(34) . This effect is all the more marked when leukocyte-depleted blood is used, and when the patient is splenectomised or in a state of functional asplenia.

Several authors recommend the use of leukoreduced blood units prior to storage which, in addition to their beneficial effect on reducing alloimmunisation, reduce transfusion reactions, refractory states to platelet and the transmission of infectious agents .(35)

With regard to the role of the spleen in the formation of allo-Ac, it is almost non-refutable that splenectomy reduces the frequency of allo-immunisation by up to 20 times in the general population(36,37) but this remains difficult to demonstrate in sickle cell patients, given the young age at which transfusions begin and the lack of knowledge of the moment when the spleen is truly non-functional, a fact which differs from one sickle cell patient to another.

2.1.4. Polymorphism of blood group antigens between donor and recipient

The polymorphism of blood group Ag between donor and recipient is one of the factors influencing alloimmunisation best documented in the literature.

The antigenic differences between the RBCs of the donor and the recipient are necessary for the initial triggering of alloimmunisation. Ac produced by the recipient is directed against Ag present on transfused RBCs. The polymorphism of these Ag varies between populations and can be a major obstacle to optimal transfusion for sickle cell patients .(39)

2.1.4.1. In populations of heterogeneous breeds

In heterogeneous populations where are differences in racial composition between donors and recipients(30,40,41) , the risk of alloimmunisation is particularly high. This is the case for Caucasian populations as blood donors and Afro-Caribbean populations as recipients. In fact, in a French study by Meunier et al.(42) , the authors showed that, in sickle cell patients living in mainland France, the risk of immunisation is increased due to the ethnic polymorphism of blood group Ag (GS), between donors, 95% of whom are of Caucasian origin, and recipients of Afro-Caribbean origin . (42)

These patients of Afro-Caribbean origin have a number of immunohaematological particularities compared with the donor population, which is Caucasian. These peculiarities are found at several levels: at the level of common Ag with different expression frequencies, particularly for Ag in the Rhesus (RH), Duffy (FY), Kidd (JK) and MNS systems, in the presence of partial or weakened variant Ag, at the level of rare phenotypes characterised by the absence of a high-frequency Ag in the RH, KEL, FY and MNS systems and at the level of low-frequency Ag in the RH and KEL systems (table I) .(43)

❖ Polymorphism of common phenotypes and antigens

The frequency of Ag D expression is 85% in the Caucasian population, and slightly higher in the Afro-Caribbean populations. The major differences concern

Ag C and Ag E, which are frequently expressed in the Caucasian population and are not expressed to any great extent in the African and West Indian populations. The Dce phenotype is the RH phenotype most frequently found in subjects of Afro-Caribbean origin (50 to 75%), whereas its frequency is less than 2% in individuals of Caucasian origin(39) . So if a sickle cell patient is transfused with blood from a Caucasian donor, the patient will be able to alloimmunise by producing an anti-C.

Other than the RH system, we find the Duffy (FY), Kidd(Jk) and MNS blood groups, for which AgFY1(Fya), JK2 (Jkb) and MNS3 (S) are frequently expressed by donors of Caucasian origin and little expressed by patients of Afro-Caribbean origin (66% vs 10% ; 74% vs 49%; 51% vs 31% respectively), hence the frequency of corresponding Ac in patients and associated post-transfusion haemolysis(43) . Thus, an Afro-Caribbean patient who is immune to a certain number of common Ags may quickly find himself in a situation where the units available are becoming increasingly rare.

❖ **Presence of partial or weakened variant antigens**

Another factor to be considered in relation to the immuno-haematological particularities of Afro-Caribbean subjects is the existence of partial or weakened variant Ag. Certain variants, rare in the Caucasian population, are frequently found in the Afro-Caribbean population and can lead to alloimmunisation.

These are partial Ags D and C, characterised by a loss of immunogenic epitopes. Patients carrying a partial C+ Ag, a frequent occurrence in the Afro-Caribbean population, may produce an anti-C directed against the non-expressed epitopes if they receive C+ RBCs from Caucasian donors(44,45) . Knowing that the production of auto-Ac is frequent in the sickle cell population(46) an anti-C associated with a partial C may be wrongly considered as an auto-Ac and would not be taken into account in the selection of RGCs(45) . Similarly, anti-D, anti-e, anti-RH18 or anti-RH34 may be easily confused with auto-Ac in sickle cell patients who are frequently alloimmunised(47,48) . This increases the risk of post-transfusion haemolytic events if these partial Ags are not identified and respected. Individuals with partial RH Ag should receive RH Ag negative RGCs.

Patients with a "weakened" variant Ag have quantitatively reduced Ag expression, but the epitopes are not systematically immunising. However, some partial variants may also have weakened expression. For many weak RH Ages, it is not known whether or not patients can become alloimmunised when exposed to the full Ag.

The elucidation of the molecular background of these HR variants in the population of African origin with more information on the incidence of Acassociated should become available .(49)

❖ **Polymorphism of rare phenotypes**

Rare erythrocyte phenotypes are characterised by the absence of expression of a high-frequency Ag (KEL: 1, -2), and by the absence of expression of all or some of the Ag common to the system (Rh null, D - -, JK: -1, -2 ...) or even by a combination of rare haplotypes in systems whose locus includes several genes (RH: -1, 2, -3, -4, 5)(50) . A certain number of rare phenotypes are found only in Afro-Caribbean populations. They are mainly described in the RH, KEL, FY and MNS systems.

*The ***best known is the FY*: -1, -2 (Fy (a- b-)) *phenotype***:

It is a rare phenotype compared with the reference donor population in mainland France. In fact, this phenotype is particularly common in the black population (almost 70%). As a general rule, transfusion of these patients does not pose any major problems because, although they may produce anti-FY1, it is exceptional for them to produce anti-FY2 or anti-FY3.

*The ***second rare phenotype encountered is the MNS*: -3, -4, -5 (S-, s-, U-) *phenotype*:***The dangerousness of the anti-MNS5 Ac is well established . (51)

Three rare specificities of the RH system are found: RH: -46 (RN phenotype; Peul origin); RH: -18 (HrS negative; Bantu origin); RH: -34 (HrB negative).

To these 3 phenotypes must be added the existence of partial RH5(e) Ag, the homozygous expression of which can lead to a transfusion impasse. Exposure to red blood cells with a common RH phenotype via transfusion or pregnancy can induce the production of anti-RH46, anti-RH18, anti-RH34 and anti-RH5 Ac respectively. In all cases, these Ac are potentially dangerous and require the use of blood units with an equivalent rare phenotype.

*Finally, *a rare phenotype found only in Afro-Caribbean populations should be mentioned: the KEL: -7 (Jsb-) phenotype.*

This poses a problem for donor recruitment, as this phenotype is not detected with commercial reagents.

❖ **Low frequency antigen polymorphism**

The last level of immuno-haematological particularities of the Afro-Caribbean populations is represented by the low frequency erythrocyte Ag or "private" Ag. A certain number of Ag are considered as "private" in the reference population of donors in metropolitan France whereas they are in fact highly prevalent in the Afro-Caribbean population. This is the case for Ag RH20 or VS(51), which is found in over 26% of black subjects and is virtually non-existent in the Caucasian population.

Similarly, KEL6 Ag (Jsa) is found in almost 20% of black subjects. Finally, there are a number of low-frequency Ag associated with partial D variants characteristic of black subjects (RH23 for DVa, RH30 for DIVa). These are rare, however, as they follow the frequency of the corresponding partial Ds.

As a rule, these "private" Ags do not pose any particular problems in a conventional transfusion context. However, they must be taken into account when the transfusion requires blood with a rare erythrocyte phenotype.

2.1.4.2. In populations of homogeneous breeds

The antigenic disparity hypothesis does not seem to be sufficiently involved in the alloimmunisation process in other populations(52,53) such as ours, which is fairly homogeneous. In patients with sickle cell disease in Uganda and Jamaica, where donors and patients are racially homogeneous, the rates of alloimmunisation were 6.1% and 2.6%(52,53) , respectively comparable to the frequencies of alloimmunisation reported for the general population of these 2 countries (1% to 6%) .(54,55)

Table II :Differences in blood groups between donors and recipients .(43)

Category	% in Caucasian donors	% among Afro-Caribbean recipients
Common antigens		
ABO Group		
A	43	27
B	9	20
O	44	49
AB	4	4
HR		
D	85	92
C	69	27
E	29	20
c	90	96
e	98	98
KEL		
K	9	2
FY		
Fy^a	66	10
Fy^b	83	23
JK		
Jk^a	77	92
Jk^b	74	49
MNS		
S	51	31
s	89	93
Partial HR antigens		
Partial D in the D+ category	1	7
Partial C among C+s	0	30
e partial among the e+	0	2
Low incidence antigens		
VS(RH20)	0,01	26-40
Jsa(KEL6)	0,01	20

Rare blood types		
U negative(MNS:-5)	0	1
Negative(HR:-18)	0	0,1
Negative HR(-34)	0	0,1
RN(RH :-46)	0	0,1
Jsbn negative (KEL:-7)	0	1

2.2. Factors linked to the recipient (specific to sickle cell disease)

Data in the literature suggest the presence of risk factors linked to the recipient, whether genetic or acquired, involved in the development of allo-Ac(23,56) . The relevance of these factors in alloimmunisation of sickle cell disease patients has not been fully elucidated.

2.2.1. Age of the recipient at the time of the first transfusions

The immune response may be influenced by the age of the sickle cell patient at the time of the first transfusions. However, results comparing the frequency of alloimmunisation in children and adults are contradictory.

Several series(7,8,23,31,57,58) have reported that the frequency of alloimmunisation decreases when transfusion treatment begins early in childhood. In a French study of a paediatric cohort of 152 children with sickle cell disease from black Africa (75%), the West Indies (18%) and North Africa (7%), the transfusion-related alloimmunisation rate was 23.4%. By contrast, in another adult cohort followed in the Île-de-France region, the post-transfusion immunisation rate was 47% .(8)

In another study carried out in the United States 29% of transfused sickle cell children developed alloAb compared with 47% of sickle cell adults(46) . Similarly, Hmida al. reported significantly higher frequencies of alloimmunisation in sickle cell patients aged between five and ten years compared with those aged under five years .(59)

Several hypotheses have been put forward to explain these findings:

- a reduced ability to produce antibodies in infants due to immunological immaturity;
- induction of immune tolerance to erythrocyte Ag by repeated early transfusions.

On the other hand, some studies have found no significant relationship between the age at which transfusion began and alloimmunisation .(8,30)

2.2.2. Sex of the recipient

We know that women have a greater potential for immunisation than men, regardless of any obstetrical history(60) . However, this notion has recently been called into question by current data on sickle cell disease.

While some studies have reported that anti-erythrocytic immunisation is more frequent in women with sickle cell disease(46) , partly explained by exposure during pregnancy(22) , others have not shown this to be the case . (8,9,21)

2.2.3. Race of recipients

The association between the risk of alloimmunisation and the race of the recipient has been clearly established.

It has been shown that black patients are more susceptible to alloimmunisation than white patients who have received a similar number of transfusions.

Elliott et al.(16) reported alloimmunisation frequencies of 30% in 107 black sickle cell patients compared with 5% in another group of white polytransfused patients consisting of 11 thalassaemics and 8 bone marrow aplasias, despite the high number of transfusions in the latter group. The authors suggest that the difference between the two groups is due to racial differences.

2.2.4. Immunogenetic factors

Alterations in regulatory T cells in alloimmunised patients, as well as abnormalities in innate immunity, have recently been implicated in the production of allo-Ac in sickle cell patients. Also found are differences in HLA class II genotype and polymorphisms in immunoregulatory genes (TRIM 21, CD81).

2.2.4.1. Type of HLA molecules and capacity to present the red cell antigen

The patient's HLA class II system is a key genetic predictor of response to RBC Ag, affecting the ability of recipients to know and present particular peptides (derived from RBC Ag). In addition, certain HLA types may be more likely to be associated with a 'responder' phenotype .(61–64)

Indeed, RBC Ag presentation has been studied in a few human studies, and it is now thought that HLA restriction exists for some erythrocyte Ag, such as Fya(63,64) and potentially Kell(65) , but not for others, in particular RH (D) . (66)

For example, in Caucasians, the formation of Ac directed against the Fya Ag is strongly associated with the DRB1 04 and DRB1 15 alleles, similar to the observations that HLA-DRB3 * 0101 and HLA-DQB1 * 0201 are the main players in alloimmunisation to HPA-1a platelet Ag.

Compared to Fya, erythrocyte KEL1 Ag is highly immunogenic, probably because potential peptides derived from KEL1 Ag can bind to multiple HLA molecules, as indicated by the wide variety of HLA II phenotypes found in individuals producing anti-KEL Ac .(63)

The HLA-DRB1 * 1503 allele has been associated with an increased risk of anti-erythrocyte alloimmunisation, regardless of the specificity of the mAb, whereas HLA-DRB1 * 0901 appears to confer protection against alloimmunisation(61) . These latest data suggest that, in addition to the direct link between HLA class II and mAb specificity, HLA alleles may also modulate alloimmunisation at a non-Ag-specific level.

2.2.4.2. Changes in the activity of regulatory T lymphocytes

Alteration of the activity of regulatory T lymphocytes (Tregs) has recently been implicated in the pathophysiology of the T response in immunised patients by affecting the response of effector Ly Th2 (T effs), which is likely to induce allo-Ac production in transfused sickle cell patients.

The identification of these interactions between T regs and T effs could in the future enable us to characterise the biomarkers associated with alloimmunisation and pave the way for new therapies to prevent anti-erythrocyte alloimmunisation (Figure 1).

❖ **Impaired regulation of effector T lymphocytes**

The stimulation of Teffs requires the interaction of peptides presented by HLA class II molecules and the TCR of circulating T lymphocytes (Figure 1). T cell activation can be modulated by Ly Th2 regulators (Tregs).

Data from mouse models indicate that Tregs inhibit the extent and frequency of alloimmunisation(67) and that alloimmunised individuals have lower Treg activity and are therefore unable to suppress Ac production compared with non-alloimmunised individuals .(68)

Possible mechanisms of Treg-mediated Ac suppression include inhibition of Ac-producing B cells(69,70) directly or indirectly via suppression of Teff function(71) . It is therefore likely that any reduction in the number or activity of Tregs will increase the likelihood of Ac production.

In humans, in a study of chronically transfused sickle cell patients, Bao et al, in 2011, found reduced peripheral Treg suppressive function and impaired Th2 response with elevated circulating interferon-gamma but low interleukin 10 compared to non-alloimmunised patients .(72)

In addition to impaired Treg function in alloimmunized sickle cell patients, Bao et al , in 2013, also found impaired activity of regulatory B cells (B regs) in these patients, particularly in their ability to inhibit the expression of pro-inflammatory cytokines by monocytes . (73)

However, it remains to be determined whether this altered immunoregulatory compartment is genetically inherited, as predicted by mathematical modelling(23) , or whether the alteration is installed only after the patient has been alloimmunised.

❖ Increased effector T lymphocyte responses

The result of a weakened immunoregulatory state is an increase in effector functions, including an increased T cell response.

In a study involving only transfused sickle cell patients(72) , we reported an altered immune response in favour of a Th2 response, these cells being known for their role in regulating humoral immunity, in the group of alloimmunised sickle cell patients. However, it remains to be determined whether these deregulations also affect other alloimmunised non-sickle cell patients.

In addition to Teffs, which are increased in alloimmunised sickle cell patients, follicular Ly Th (Tfh), particularly those expressing TIGIT (T-cell immunoreceptor with immunoglobulin and immunoreceptor tyrosine based inhibitory domains)(Tfh TIGIT+),key effector cells specialised in cooperating with B lymphocytes to induce the primary Ac response, as well as supporting the differentiation of B lymphocytes into Ac-producing B cells(74) are increased.

Godefry et al(74) , suggest that although TIGIT+ Tfh frequencies and TIGIT expression levels per cell were comparable between allo and non-allo sickle cell patients, TfhTIGIT+ from alloimmunised patients secrete more IL-21 and express more B-cell costimulatory markers, such as inducible T cell co-stimulator (ICOS) and CD40 ligand (CD40L) (Figure 2);ICOSand CD40 ligand (CD40L) (Figure 2). This was explained by increased TIGIT signalling in alloimmunised patients or conversely by a deficiency in TIGIT-mediated responses and signalling pathways in non-alloimmunised patients.

Further studies are currently underway to characterise the differences in TIGIT-mediated responses between allo- and non-alloimmunised sickle cell patients in order to identify potential biomarkers associated with TfhTIGIT+(24) . These studies will serve as an aid to the development targeted therapeutic strategies based on TfhTIGIT+ inhibition.

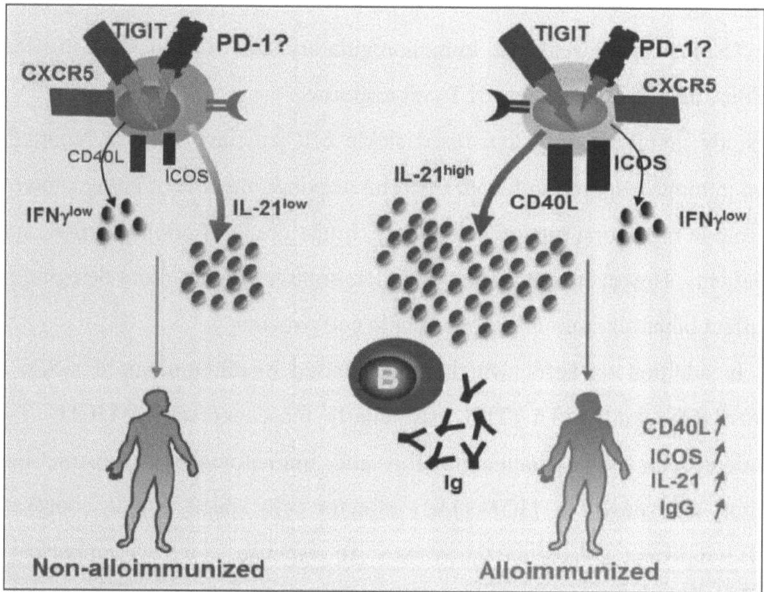

Figure2 : Differences in Tfh TIGIT+ activity between allo and non-allo sickle cell patients .(24)

The data suggest that alloimmunised sickle cell patients have comparable levels of TIGIT receptors and frequencies of TIGIT+ Tfh with non-alloimmunised patients. However, the functional activity of Tfhs differed between the 2 groups: TIGIT+ Tfhs from non-alloimmunised sickle cell patients expressed fewer B cell costimulatory markers (inducible T cell co-stimulator (ICOS) and CD40 ligand (CD40L)) and produced less IL-21; this was explained by differences in TIGIT receptor signalling between the 2 groups. As a result, non-alloimmunised sickle cell Tfh are less effective in helping B lymphocytes to produce IgG compared with alloimmunised sickle cell patients who have more potent TfhTIGIT+.

2.2.4.3. Polymorphism of immunoregulatory elements (TRIM 21,CD81)

The literature suggests that polymorphisms in immunoregulatory genes may also influence anti-erythrocyte alloimmunisation in sickle cell disease.

For example, the polymorphism of TRIM 21, an immunoregulatory gene close to the ß-globin gene, and also its molecular expression Ro52 have recently been shown to be associated with an increase in the alloimmunisation rate in sickle cell patients, particularly in early childhood .(23)

Another study of SNPs (single nucleotide polymorphisms) in alloimmunised and non-alloimmunised sickle cell patients implicated CD81 polymorphisms as contributors to recipient immune responses by modulating B cell activity and disrupting dendritic cell function .(75)

Recently, a study published in 2019 of 19 SNPs from allo and non-alloimmunized sickle cell patients identified a higher risk of alloimmunization for SNPs in the TLR1/TANK and MALT genes compared to those in the STAM / IFNAR1 and STAT4 genes .(76)

2.2.5. Inflammatory state of sickle cell disease

A key feature of sickle cell disease is the persistence of a chronic inflammatory state, even in a stable state.

Studies in murines -(68,8082) and in humans -(8386) have shown that in inflammatory situations Ac are produced more often and at higher levels, via pro-inflammatory cytokines.

In humans, other studies have investigated the impact of different types of inflammatory conditions on anti-erythrocyte alloimmunisation: one suggested that the occurrence of febrile transfusion reactions may be associated with subsequent allo-Ac formation(84) , another showed that inflammatory bowel disease may be a risk factor for allo-immunisation(85) and another reported that transfusion at the time of an acute inflammatory episode (such as an acute chest syndrome, or a vaso-occlusive crisis) may be more likely to result in allo-Ac formation than transfusion in the absence of acute illness(86) .

2.2.6. Role of haemolysis in alloimmunisation

The chronic haemolysis found in sickle cell disease is increasingly accepted as a factor involved in the alloimmunisation process via an enzyme: haem oxygenase 1 (HO-1). However, prospective studies are underway to determine whether the drop in HO-1 is a precursor to alloimmunisation or conversely whether alloimmunisation leads to a drop in HO-1 levels.

In the physiological state, haemolysis of RBCs leads to a significant release of haemoglobin and its oxidised form, haem, into the circulation(87,88) . Through its enzymatic activity, HO-1 degrades haem into bilirubin, carbon monoxide and iron, thus conferring cyto-protective and anti-inflammatory effects by reducing the availability of intracellular haem . (89,90)

In an alloimmunised sickle cell patient, low levels of HO-1 in monocytes and macrophages in the liver and spleen lead to inefficient elimination of haem after RBC transfusion, resulting in a pro-inflammatory state (high levels of IL-12) that stimulates proliferation of effector Ly T cells while inhibiting the development of Treg cells, thereby increasing the likelihood of alloAC development by B lymphocytes (Figure 3).

On the other hand, the efficient elimination of haem in non-alloimmunised patients ensures an immunoregulatory and anti-inflammatory state (low levels of IL-12 resulting in an expansion of Tregs and a reduction in Teffs) which is less favourable to alloimmunisation .(91,92)

In line with the latter data, Fasano et al(86) found that transfusion of RGCs to already alloimmunised patients under acute conditions associated with increased haemolysis such as an acute chest syndrome or vaso-occlusive crisis leads to the formation of new anti-erythrocyte alloAs.

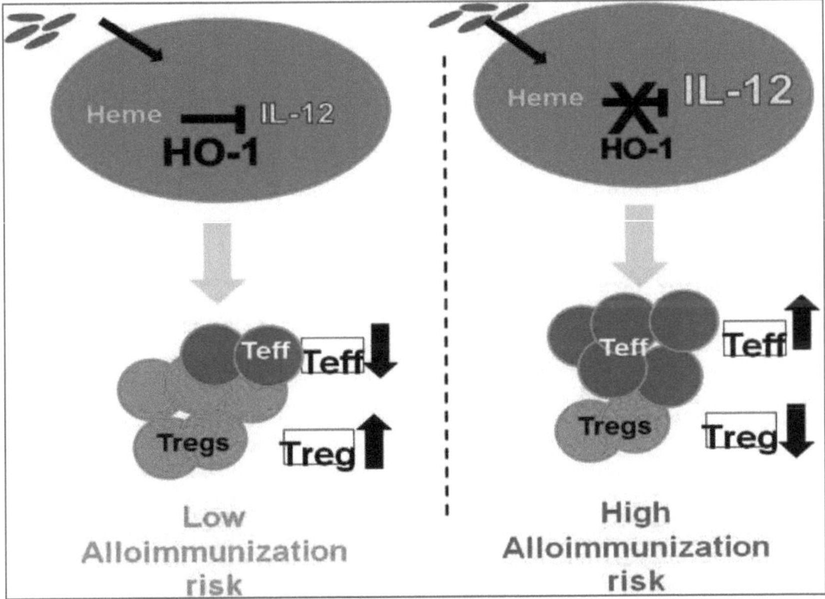

Figure3 : Levels and activity of HO-1 in the innate immune cells of sickle cell disease patients in response to haemolysis .(24)

Sickle cell patients with a high concentration of HO-1 effectively inhibit the pro-inflammatory cytokine IL-12 in response to the presence of extracellular free haem. This results in a high Treg/T effplus ratio, which in turn suppresses B cell responses and reduces their risk of alloimmunisation. In contrast, low HO-1 levels or activity will lead to an inability to buffer IL-12, lowering the Treg/T eff ratio and increasing the risk of alloimmunisation.

3. Transfusion management strategies to prevent alloimmunisation and delayed haemolysis

3.1 Transfusion rules for patients with sickle cell disease

- As soon as sickle cell anaemia has been diagnosed, it is recommended that, wherever possible, the following work-up is carried out before any transfusion. This assessment should include:

- determination of ABO RH-KEL blood groups. In France, RH-KEL1 erythrocyte phenotyping is indicated for sickle cell disease patients who are polytransfused ,(93)

- pre-transfusion irregular agglutinin test (RAI),

- phenotyping extended to the systems most commonly involved in immunisation (Duffy, Kidd, MNS systems) to take account of the common immunogenic Ag of these systems.

The practice of the extended phenotype varies from one country to another: in France, the extended phenotype is prescribed as soon as an alloimmunisation develops.

The usefulness and cost-effectiveness of early extended phenotyping has not been reported, despite the fact that it can save valuable time in the transfusion management of patients with multiple allo- and auto-As in acute situations.

Molecular tools are already available for genotyping common Ag as well as variant antigens and rare GS. Such tools are increasingly used in reference laboratories. With advances in genomics technology, high-throughput DNA typing platforms will become less expensive for donor typing and should reduce the need for rare serological reagents to find rare compatible donors . (94)

- The type of blood products prescribed depends on the RAI. For patients with

Non-immunised (negative IRA on the day of transfusion and in the history), the RGCs delivered are phenotyped Rhesus (D, C, E, c, e) and KEL 1 and counted in the laboratory.

Prior to transfusion, a positive identification or positivity in the IAA history should lead to the phenotype of transfused red cell concentrates being extended to immunogenic GS systems beyond the Rhesus Kell systems, i.e. the Kidd, Duffy and MNS systems. Individuals with partial Rh Ag should receive RBCs without these Ag.

Figure 4 illustrates an algorithm describing the recommended transfusion strategy for patients with sickle cell disease.

- If there is a history of post-transfusion haemolysis or
transfusion inefficiency, complex alloimmunisation or poly alloimmunisation, transfusion indications should be restricted to life-threatening situations (26). Rationalisation of transfusion indications in sickle cell disease patients is still recommended . (95)

- In addition, it is important to take HLA and alloimmunisation associations into account, so that the units to be transfused for polytransfused patients can be selected taking into account their antigenic susceptibilities.

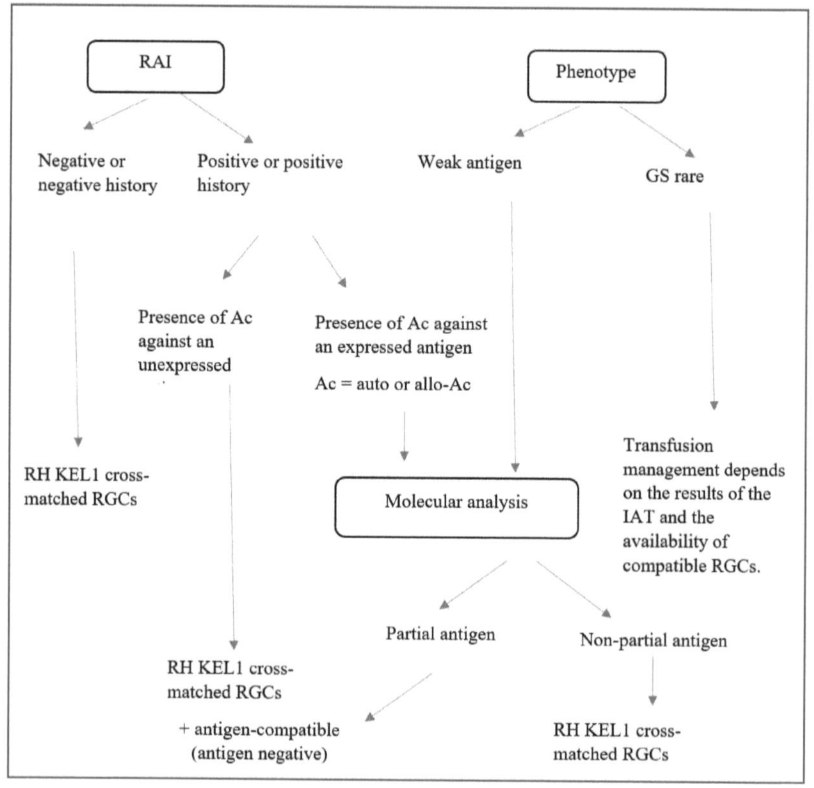

Figure4 : Algorithm of the recommended transfusion strategy for patients with sickle cell disease.

All recommendations are based on the results of irregular agglutinin (RAI) tests and the patient's extended phenotype. *For patients with no detectable antibodies*, no known previous antibodies (Ac) and no abnormal erythrocyte phenotype, it is recommended to use RGCs phenotypedRH-KEL1, leucocyte-depleted and matched. When Ac is identified or known in the patient's history, 2 scenarios may be encountered: (1) The corresponding antigen (Ag) is not expressed on the patient's red blood cells (RBCs); consequently, the Ac is an allo-Ac, and therefore RBCs lacking the corresponding Ag will be transfused.(2) The corresponding Ag is expressed on the patient's RBCs, and serological and/or molecular studies are required to determine whether the Ac is unallo-Ac produced against a partial Ag or an auto-Ac. If it is an allo-Ac, the RBCs must be RH-KEL1 phenotyped and matched. In the case of an auto-Ac, compatibility with the corresponding Ag is not necessary. *For the patient's phenotype*, 2 situations must be considered: (1) Presence of a weak Ag, where molecular analysis will be required to determine whether it is a partial Ag. If the patient has no detectable Ag, transfusion with a negative antigenic unit is preferred, although positive antigenic RBCs may also be delivered as the risk of alloimmunisation in patients with weak Ag has not yet been determined. (2) Another situation is the presence of a rare phenotype. Transfusion management of these patients is extremely difficult due to the lack of immediate availability of pheno-compatible blood units: autologous transfusion, ABO- and pheno-compatible sibling blood, rare phenotype blood bank.

3.2. Prospects for therapeutic strategies to prevent alloimmunisation and delayed haemolysis

Ongoing studies should explore new approaches to inhibiting alloimmunisation in sickle cell disease. Immunomodulatory therapies, such as the use of immune cell depressants, costimulatory blockade and cytokine blockade, may be effective in suppressing alloimmunisation (Figure 1), although their use should be cautious given the risk of infection in sickle cell patients.

Rituximab, a chimeric mouse anti-human monoclonal antibody which binds to CD20 expressed on all B cells, has been used successfully to treat autoAb production and haemolysis in sickle cell disease(96,97) by depleting pathogenic Ac-producing B cells(54) . Could it also be effective in cases of alloimmunisation?

Blocking TNF (Tumor Necrosis Factor) using anti-TNF neutralizing Acα , has recently been shown to inhibit alloimmunization in a transplant model(98) . TNF inhibition has anti-inflammatory effects on multiple pathways, including endothelial activation and leukocyte recruitment, known to be involved in vaso-occlusive crises(99,100) and may therefore be effective in sickle cell disease for the suppression of alloimmunisation.

Similarly, adenosine 2A receptor agonists have been shown to be effective in treating pulmonary inflammation and vaso-occlusive crises in sickle cell mice by inhibiting the activation of a variant of NK cells and other leukocytes(101) and may represent an alternative strategy for limiting alloimmunisation by down-regulating lymphocyte activation.

Blocking co-stimulatory interactions between Ly T and B, for example, by inhibiting the CD40-CD40 ligand pathway with an anti CD40 ligand monoclonal Ac or the B7 pathway with CTLA-4Ig / Abatacept(102) are other possible options.

Finally, tolerance induction using immunodominant peptides derived from immunogenic polypeptides(103) or Treg immunotherapy(67) have shown their feasibility in mouse studies to inhibit allo-Ac production, some of which are being actively pursued as additional therapeutic approaches for the prevention of allo-immunisation.

Conclusion

Anti-erythrocyte alloimmunisation is a serious problem in polytransfused sickle cell patients, particularly in view of the increasing longevity of patients and the growing number of transfusion indications in the management of these patients.

Although the factors influencing the occurrence of alloimmunisation are still largely unknown, published studies point to both genetic and non-genetic factors.

Challenges remain in the diagnosis, prevention and management of alloimmunisation in sickle cell disease. Understanding the mechanisms and associated risk factors will help to develop strategies to prevent and inhibit Ac production in transfused patients and to preserve the potentially life-threatening prognosis.

Studies on mouse models are underway to explain the molecular immune mechanisms involved in alloimmunisation.

At the same time, careful epidemiological and prospective studies are needed to investigate critical issues, including the optimal age for initial exposure to RBC antigens. Ongoing studies should clarify the role of genetic factors in alloimmunisation and help identify susceptibility genes that contribute to alloimmunisation.

For the transfusion management of patients with sickle cell disease, a review of the transfusion policy to be undertaken in our country should take account of the resources available.

References

REFERENCES

1. WHO | Global epidemiology of haemoglobin disorders and related service indicators. WHO. Available at: https://www.who.int/bulletin/volumes/86/6/06-036673-ab/fr/

2. R.Hafsia.Evaluation of iron overload during sickle cell disease: about 94 cases. Tunis Med. 2011; vol 89 (n°6):548-552.

3. Galactéros F. [Sickle cell disease pathophysiology: from theoretical to practical aspects]. Rev Prat. Sept 2004;54(14):1534-42.

4. Walter PB, Harmatz P, Vichinsky E. Iron metabolism and iron chelation in sickle cell disease. Acta Haematol. 2009;122(2-3):174-83.

5. Wanko SO, Telen MJ. Transfusion management in sickle cell disease. Hematol Oncol Clin North Am. Oct 2005;19(5):803-26, v-vi.

6. Lefrère JJ, Schvec JF. Transfusion in haematology. Montrouge: John LibbeyEurotext; 2010.

6. Win N, New H, Lee E, de la Fuente J. Hyperhemolysissyndrom in sicklecelldisease: case report (recurrentepisode) and literaturereview. Transfusion 2008;48:1231-8.

7. Pham B-N, Le Pennec P-Y, Rouger P. Anti-erythrocyte alloimmunisation. Transfus Clin Biol. Dec 2012;19(6):321-32.

8. Ben Amor I, Louati N, Khemekhem H, Dhieb A, Rekik H, Mdhaffar M, et al. Anti-erythrocyte immunisation in haemoglobinopathies: 84 cases. Transfus Clin Biol. Dec 2012;19(6):345-52.

9. Salah NB et al. Anti-erythrocyte and anti-HLA immunization during hemoglobinopathies. Transfus Clin Biol. 2014

10. Orlina AR, Unger PJ, Koshy M. Post-transfusion alloimmunization in patients with sickle cell disease. Am. J. Hematol. 1978;5(2):101-6.

11. Spanos T, Karageorga M, Ladis V, Peristeri J, Hatziliami A, Kattamis C. Red cell alloantibodies in patients with thalassemia. Vox Sang. 1990;58(1):50-5.

12. Mintz PD. Alloimmunization to red blood cell antigens by transfusion. Blood. May 2010;115(21):4315; author reply 4315-4316.

13. Ambruso DR, Githens JH, Alcorn R, Dixon DJ, Brown LJ, Vaughn WM, et al. Experience with donors matched for minor blood group antigens in patients with sickle cell anemia who are receiving chronic transfusion therapy. TRANSFUSION. Feb 1987;27(1):94-8.

14. Coles SM, Klein HG, Holland PV. Alloimmunization in two multitransfused patient populations. TRANSFUSION. August 1981;21(4):462-6.

15. Blumberg N, Ross K, Avila E, Peck K. Should chronic transfusions be matched for antigens other than ABO and Rho(D)? Vox Sang. 1984;47(3):205-8.

16. Vichinsky EP, Earles A, Johnson RA, Hoag MS, Williams A, Lubin B. Alloimmunization in sickle cell anemia and transfusion of racially unmatched blood. NEJM. June 1990;322(23):1617-21.

17. Bauer MP, Wiersum-Osselton J, Schipperus M, Vandenbroucke JP, Briët E. Clinical predictors of alloimmunization after red blood cell transfusion. TRANSFUSION. Nov 2007;47(11):2066-71.

18. Rosse WF, Gallagher D, Kinney TR, Castro O, Dosik H, Moohr J, et al. Transfusion and alloimmunization in sickle cell disease. The Cooperative Study of Sickle Cell Disease. Blood. Oct 1990; 76(7):1431-7.

19. Sarnaik S, Schornack J, Lusher JM. The incidence of development of irregular red cell antibodies in patients with sickle cell anemia. TRANSFUSION. June 1986;26(3):249-52.

20. Cox JV, Steane E, Cunningham G, Frenkel EP. Risk of alloimmunization and delayed hemolytic transfusion reactions in patients with sickle cell disease. Arch Intern Med. Nov 1988;148(11):2485-9.

21. Murao M, Viana MB. Risk factors for alloimmunization by patients with sickle cell disease. Braz J Med Biol Res. May 2005;38(5):675-82.

22. Schonewille H, van de Watering LMG, Loomans DSE, Brand A. Red blood cell alloantibodies after transfusion: factors influencing incidence and specificity. TRANSFUSION. Feb 2006;46(2):250-6.

23. Higgins JM, Sloan SR. Stochastic modeling of human RBC alloimmunization: evidence for a distinct population of immunologic responders. Blood. Sept 2008;112(6):2546-53.

24. Yazdanbakhsh K. Immunoregulatory networks in sickle cell alloimmunization. HEMATOL-AM SOC HEMATDec 2016;2016(1):457-61.

25. Yazdanbakhsh K, Ware RE, Noizart-Pirenne F. Red blood cell alloimmunization in sickle cell disease: pathophysiology, risk factors, and transfusion management. Blood. Juil 2012; 120(3):528-37.

26. Norol F, Nadjahi J, Bachir D, Desaint C, Guillou Bataille M, Beaujean F, et al. Transfusion and alloimmunisation in sickle cell patients. Transfus Clin Biol. Jan 1994;1(1):27-34.

27. Godfrey GJ, Lockwood W, Kong M, Bertolone S, Raj A. Antibody development in pediatric sickle cell patients undergoing erythrocytapheresis. Pediatr Blood Cancer. Dec 2010;55(6):1134-7.

28. Castro O, Sandler SG, Houston-Yu P, Rana S. Predicting the effect of transfusing only phenotype-matched RBCs to patients with sickle cell disease: theoretical and practical implications. TRANSFUSION 2002;42:684-90.

29. Shaz BH, Zimring JC, Demmons DG, Hillyer CD. Blood donation and blood transfusion: special considerations for African Americans. Transfus Med Rev. 2008 Jul;22(3):202-14.

30. Moreira Júnior G, Bordin JO, Kuroda A, Kerbauy J. Red blood cell alloimmunization in sickle cell disease: the influence of racial and antigenic pattern differences between donors and recipients in Brazil. Am J Hematol. July 1996;52(3):197-200.

31. Gader AGMA, Al Ghumlas AK, Al-Momen AKM. Transfusion medicine in a developing country - Alloantibodies to red blood cells in multi-transfused patients in Saudi Arabia. Transfus apher sci. Dec 2008;39(3):199-204.

32. Davies SC, Roberts-Harewood M. Blood transfusion in sickle cell disease. Blood Reviews. June 1997;11(2):57-71.

33. Joep W. R. Sins, David J. Mager, Shyrin C. A. T. Davis et al . Pharmacotherapeutic strategies in the prevention of acute, vaso-occlusive pain in sickle cell disease: a systematic review. Blood. Adv. 2017 Aug 22; 1(19): 1598-1616.

34. Silvy M, Tournamille C, Babinet J, Pakdaman S, Cohen S, Chiaroni J, et al. Red blood cell immunization in sickle cell disease: evidence of a large responder group and a low rate of anti-Rh linked to partial Rh phenotype. Haematologica. Jul 2014;99(7):e115-7.

35. Singer ST, Wu V, Mignacca R, Kuypers FA, Morel P, Vichinsky EP. Alloimmunization and erythrocyte autoimmunization in transfusion-dependent thalassemia patients of predominantly Asian descent. Blood. Nov 2000;96(10):3369-73.

36. Ameen R, Al-Shemmari S, Al-Humood S, Chowdhury RI, Al-Eyaadi O, Al-Bashir A. RBC alloimmunization and autoimmunization among transfusion-dependent Arab thalassemia patients. TRANSFUSION. Nov 2003;43(11):1604-10.

37. Hendrickson JE, Roback JD, Hillyer CD, Zimring JC. An Intact Spleen Is Required for Alloimmunization to Transfused Red Blood Cells Due to Intrasplenic Activation of CD4+ T Cells. Blood. Nov 2007;110(11):453-453.

38. Evers D, van der Bom JG, Tijmensen J, de Haas M, Middelburg RA, de Vooght KMK, et al. Absence of the spleen and the occurrence of primary red cell alloimmunization in humans. Haematologica. August 2017;102(8):e289-92.

39. Noizat-Pirenne F. [Immunohematologic characteristics in the Afro-caribbean population. Consequences for transfusion safety]. Transfus Clin Biol. June 2003;10(3):185-91.

40. Noizat-Pirenne F. Immunohaematological particularities in African and West Indian populations. Transfu clin biol. May 2003;10:185-91.

41. Vichinsky EP, Luban NL, Wright E, Olivieri N, Driscoll C, Pegelow CH, et al. Prospective RBC phenotype matching in a stroke-prevention trial in sickle cell anemia: a multicenter transfusion trial. TRANSFUSION. Sept 2001;41(9):1086-92.

42. Luban NL. Variability in rates of alloimmunization in different groups of children with sickle cell disease: effect of ethnic background. Am J Pediatr Hematol Oncol. 1989;11(3):314-9.

43. Meunier N, Rodet M, Bonin P, Chadebech P, Chami B, Lee K, et al. Study of a cohort of 206 transfused adult sickle cell patients: immunisation, transfusion risk and resources of packed red blood cells. Transfus clin biol.Dec 2008;15(6):377-82.

44. The Blood Group Antigen FactsBook - 3rd Edition. Available at: https://www.elsevier.com/books/the-blood-group-antigen-factsbook/reid/978-0-12-415849-8

45. Flegel WA, Wagner FF. Molecular genetics of RH. Vox Sang. 2000;78 Suppl 2:109-15.

46. Tournamille C, Meunier-Costes N, Costes B, Martret J, Barrault A, Gauthier P, et al. Partial C antigen in sickle cell disease patients: clinical relevance and prevention of alloimmunization. TRANSFUSION. Jan 2010;50(1):13-9.

47. Aygun B, Padmanabhan S, Paley C, Chandrasekaran V. Clinical significance of RBC alloantibodies and autoantibodies in sickle cell patients who received transfusions. TRANSFUSION. Jan 2002;42(1):37-43.

48. Lomas-Francis C, Yomtovian R, McGrath C, Walker PS, Reid ME. A confusion in antibody identification: anti-D production after anti-hrB. Immunohematology. 2007;23(4):158-60.

49. Noizat-Pirenne F, Lee K, Pennec P-YL, Simon P, Kazup P, Bachir D, et al. Rare RHCE phenotypes in black individuals of Afro-Caribbean origin: identification and transfusion safety. Blood. Dec 2002;100(12):4223-31.

50. Noizat-Pirenne F, Tournamille C. Relevance of RH variants in transfusion of sickle cell patients.Transfus Clin Biol. 2011;18(5):527-535)

51. Giblett ER. A Critique of the Theoretical Hazard of Inter vs. Intra-Racial Transfusion*. TRANSFUSION. 1961;1(4):233-8.

52. Storry JR. Human blood groups: inheritance and importance in transfusion medicine. J Infus Nurs. Dec 2003;26(6):367-72.

53. Natukunda B, Schonewille H, Ndugwa C, Brand A. Red blood cell alloimmunization in sickle cell disease patients in Uganda. TRANSFUSION. Jan 2010;50(1):20-5.

54. Olujohungbe A, Hambleton I, Stephens L, Serjeant B, Serjeant G. Red cell antibodies in patients with homozygous sickle cell disease: a comparison of patients in Jamaica and the United Kingdom. Br J Haematol. June 2001;113(3):661-5.

55. Noizat-Pirenne F, Bachir D, Chadebech P, Michel M, Plonquet A, Lecron J-C, et al. Rituximab for prevention of delayed hemolytic transfusion reaction in sickle cell disease. Haematologica. Dec 2007;92(12):e132-135.

56. Natukunda B, Brand A, Schonewille H. Red blood cell alloimmunization from an African perspective. Curr Opin Hematol. Nov 2010;17(6):565-70.

57. Hendrickson JE, Tormey CA, Shaz BH. Red blood cell alloimmunization mitigation strategies. Transfus Med Rev. Jul 2014;28(3):137-44.

58. Gill FM, Sleeper LA, Weiner SJ, Brown AK, Bellevue R, Grover R, et al. Clinical events in the first decade in a cohort of infants with sickle cell

disease. Cooperative Study of Sickle Cell Disease. Blood. July 1995;86(2):776-83.

59. Verduzco LA, Nathan DG. Sickle cell disease and stroke. Blood. Dec 2009;114(25):5117-25.

60. Hmida S, Mojaat N, Maamar M, Bejaoui M, Mediouni M, Boukef K. Red cell alloantibodies in patients with haemoglobinopathies. Nouv Rev Fr Hematol. Oct 1994;36(5):363-6.

61. Rouger P, Salmon C. La pratique des allo et auto-anticorps anti-érythrocytes. Paris: Masson; 1981.

62. Hoppe C, Klitz W, Vichinsky E, Styles L. HLA type and risk of alloimmunization in sickle cell disease. Am. J. Hematol. 2009;84(7):462-4.

63. Schonewille H, Doxiadis IIN, Levering WHBM, Roelen DL, Claas FHJ, Brand A. HLA-DRB1 associations in individuals with single and multiple clinically relevant red blood cell antibodies. TRANSFUSION. August 2014;54(8):1971-80.

64. Noizat-Pirenne F, Tournamille C, Bierling P, Roudot-Thoraval F, Le Pennec P-Y, Rouger P, et al. Relative immunogenicity of Fya and K antigens in a Caucasian population, based on HLA class II restriction analysis. TRANSFUSION. August 2006;46(8):1328-33.

65. Picard C, Frassati C, Basire A, Buhler S, Galicher V, Ferrera V, et al. Positive association of DRB1 04 and DRB1 15 alleles with Fya immunization in a Southern European population. TRANSFUSION. Nov 2009;49(11):2412-7.

66. Stephen J, Cairns LS, Pickford WJ, Vickers MA, Urbaniak SJ, Barker RN. Identification, immunomodulatory activity, and immunogenicity of the major helper T-cell epitope on the K blood group antigen. Blood. June 2012;119(23):5563-74.

67. Brantley SG, Ramsey G. Red cell alloimmunization in multitransfused HLA-typed patients. TRANSFUSION. Oct 1988;28(5):463-6.

68. Yu J, Heck S, Yazdanbakhsh K. Prevention of red cell alloimmunization by CD25 regulatory T cells in mouse models. Am J Hematol. August 2007;82(8):691-6.

69. Bao W, Yu J, Heck S, Yazdanbakhsh K. Regulatory T-cell status in red cell alloimmunized responder and nonresponder mice. Blood. May 2009;113(22):5624-7.

70. Iikuni N, Lourenço EV, Hahn BH, La Cava A. Cutting edge: Regulatory T cells directly suppress B cells in systemic lupus erythematosus. J Immunol. August 2009;183(3):1518-22.

71. Lim HW, Hillsamer P, Banham AH, Kim CH. Cutting edge: direct suppression of B cells by CD4+ CD25+ regulatory T cells. J Immunol. Oct 2005;175(7):4180-3.

72. Wing JB, Sakaguchi S. Multiple treg suppressive modules and their adaptability. Front Immunol. 2012;3:178.

73. Bao W, Zhong H, Li X, Lee MT, Schwartz J, Sheth S, et al. Immune regulation in chronically transfused allo-antibody responder and nonresponder patients with sickle cell disease and β-thalassemia major. Am J Hematol. Dec 2011;86(12):1001-6.

74. Bao W, Zhong H, Manwani D, Vasovic L, Uehlinger J, Lee MT, et al. Regulatory B cell Compartment in Transfused Alloimmunized and Non-alloimmunized Patients with Sickle Cell Disease. Am J Hematol. Sept 2013;88(9):736-40.

75. Godefroy E, Zhong H, Pham P, Friedman D, Yazdanbakhsh K. TIGIT-positive circulating follicular helper T cells display robust B-cell help functions: potential role in sickle cell alloimmunization. Haematologica. Nov 2015;100(11):1415-25.

76. Tatari-Calderone Z, Tamouza R, Le Bouder GP, Dewan R, Luban NLC, Lasserre J, et al. The Association of CD81 Polymorphisms with Alloimmunization in Sickle Cell Disease. Clin Dev Immunol;2013.

77. Meinderts SM, Gerritsma JJ, Sins JWR, de Boer M, van Leeuwen K, Biemond BJ, et al. Identification of genetic biomarkers for alloimmunization in sickle cell disease. Br J Haematol. Sept 2019;186(6):887-99.

78. Hendrickson JE, Chadwick TE, Roback JD, Hillyer CD, Zimring JC. Inflammation enhances consumption and presentation of transfused RBC antigens by dendritic cells. Blood. Oct 2007;110(7):2736-43.

79. Trombetta ES, Mellman I. Cell biology of antigen processing in vitro and in vivo. Annu Rev Immunol. 2005;23:975-1028.

80. Hendrickson JE, Hod EA, Perry JR, Ghosh S, Chappa P, Adisa O, et al. Alloimmunization to transfused HOD red blood cells is not increased in mice with sickle cell disease. TRANSFUSION. Feb 2012;52(2):231-40.

81. Hibbert JM, Hsu LL, Bhathena SJ, Irune I, Sarfo B, Creary MS, et al. Proinflammatory cytokines and the hypermetabolism of children with sickle cell disease. Exp Biol Med Jan 2005;230(1):68-74.

82. Bourantas KL, Dalekos GN, Makis A, Chaidos A, Tsiara S, Mavridis A. Acute phase proteins and interleukins in steady state sickle cell disease. Eur J Haematol. July 1998;61(1):49-54.

83. Jison ML, Munson PJ, Barb JJ, Suffredini AF, Talwar S, Logun C, et al. Blood mononuclear cell gene expression profiles characterize the oxidant, hemolytic, and inflammatory stress of sickle cell disease. Blood. Juill 2004;104(1):270-80.

84. Platt OS. Sickle cell anemia as an inflammatory disease. J Clin Invest. August 2000;106(3):337-8.

85. Yazer MH, Triulzi DJ, Shaz B, Kraus T, Zimring JC. Does a febrile reaction to platelets predispose recipients to red blood cell alloimmunization? TRANSFUSION. June 2009;49(6):1070-5.

86. Papay P, Hackner K, Vogelsang H, Novacek G, Primas C, Reinisch W, et al. High risk of transfusion-induced alloimmunization of patients with inflammatory bowel disease. Am J Med. Jul 2012;125(7):717.e1-8.

87. Fasano RM, Booth GS, Miles M, Du L, Koyama T, Meier ER, et al. Red blood cell alloimmunization is influenced by recipient inflammatory state at time of transfusion in patients with sickle cell disease. Br J Haematol. Jan 2015;168(2):291-300.

88. Lezcano NE, Odo N, Kutlar A, Brambilla D, Adams RJ. Regular transfusion lowers plasma free hemoglobin in children with sickle-cell disease at risk for stroke. STROKE. June 2006;37(6):1424-6.

89. Reiter CD, Wang X, Tanus-Santos JE, Hogg N, Cannon RO, Schechter AN, et al. Cell-free haemoglobin limits nitric oxide bioavailability in sickle-cell disease. Nat Med. Dec 2002;8(12):1383-9.

90. Ryter SW, Alam J, Choi AMK. Heme oxygenase-1/carbon monoxide: from basic science to therapeutic applications. Physiol Rev. Apr 2006;86(2):583-650.

91. Nath KA, Balla G, Vercellotti GM, Balla J, Jacob HS, Levitt MD, et al. Induction of heme oxygenase is a rapid, protective response in rhabdomyolysis in the rat. J Clin Invest. July 1992;90(1):267-70.

92. Zhong H, Bao W, Friedman D, Yazdanbakhsh K. Hemin controls T cell polarization in sickle cell alloimmunization. J Immunol. Jul 2014;193(1):102-10.

93. Zhong H, Yazdanbakhsh K. Differential control of Helios(+/-) Treg development by monocyte subsets through disparate inflammatory cytokines. Blood. March 2013;121(13):2494-502.

94. CircularN°32/15 of 11 May 2015, relating to transfusion safety(Ministry of Public Health of the Republic of Tunisia).

95. Anstee DJ. Red cell genotyping and the future of pretransfusion testing. Blood. 9 Jul 2009; 114(2):248-56.

96. Rodrigues C, Sell AM, Guelsin GAS et al. HLA polymorphisms and risk of red blood cell alloimmunisation in polytransfused patients with sickle cell anaemia.Transfus Med.2017 Dec;27(6):437-443.

97. Bachmeyer C, Maury J, Parrot A, et al. Rituximab as an effective treatment of hyperhemolysis syndrome in sicklecellanemia. *Am J Hematol.* 2010;85(1):91-92.

98. Reff ME, Carner K, Chambers KS, et al. Depletion of B cells in vivo by a chimeric mouse human monoclonal antibody to CD20. Blood.1994;83(2):435-445.)

99. FrancoSalinas G, Mai HL, Jovanovic V, et al. TNF blockadeabrogates the induction of T cell dependent humoral responses in an allotransplantation model. J LeukocBiol. 2011;90(2):367-375.).

100 Turhan A, Weiss LA, Mohandas N, Coller BS, Frenette PS. Primaryrole for adherent leukocytes in sickle cell vascular occlusion: a new paradigm.ProcNatlAcadSci U S A. 2002;99(5):3047-3051.

101. Tracey D, Klareskog L, Sasso EH, Salfeld JG,Tak PP. Tumor necrosis factor antagonist mechanisms of action: a comprehensive review. PharmacolTher. 2008;117(2):244-279.

102 Wallace KL, Linden J. Adenosine A2A receptors induced on iNKT and NK cells reduce pulmonary inflammation and injury in mice with sickle cell disease. *Blood.* 2010;116 (23):5010-5020.

103. Ford ML, Larsen CP.Translating costimulation blockade to the clinic: lessons learned from three pathways. ImmunolRev. 2009;229 (1):294-306.

104. Hall AM, Cairns LS, Altmann DM, Barker RN, Urbaniak SJ. Immune responses and tolerance to the RhDblood group protein in HLA-transgenicmice. *Blood.* 2005;105(5):2175-2179.

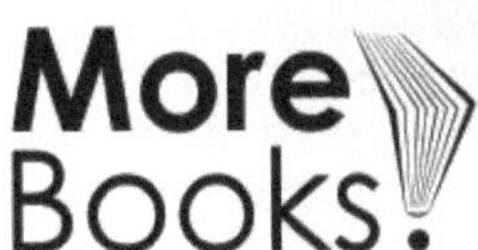

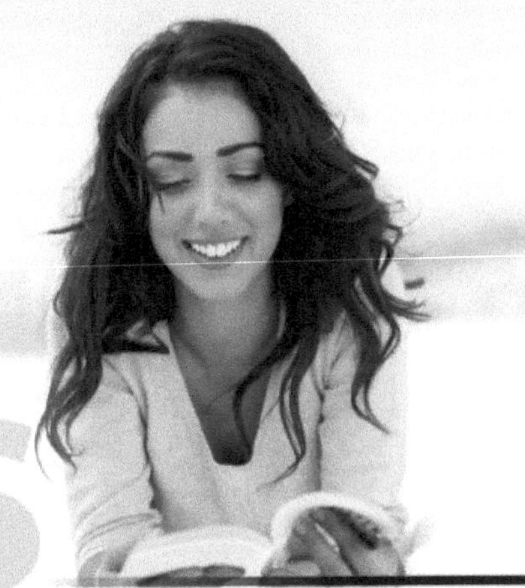

yes
I want morebooks!

Buy your books fast and straightforward online - at one of world's fastest growing online book stores! Environmentally sound due to Print-on-Demand technologies.

Buy your books online at
www.morebooks.shop

Kaufen Sie Ihre Bücher schnell und unkompliziert online – auf einer der am schnellsten wachsenden Buchhandelsplattformen weltweit! Dank Print-On-Demand umwelt- und ressourcenschonend produziert.

Bücher schneller online kaufen
www.morebooks.shop

info@omniscriptum.com
www.omniscriptum.com

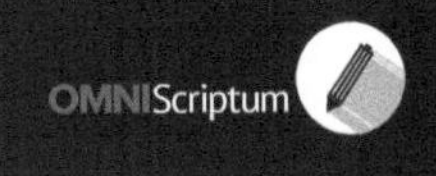

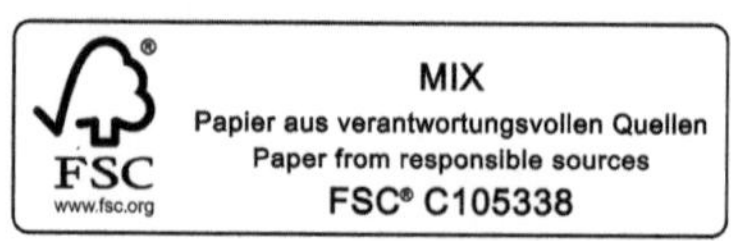

Printed by Books on Demand GmbH, Norderstedt / Germany